Is Tommy

Ok

Or

Not Ok?

Written by Jennifer Cameron

Hi! My name is Tommy and I am 6 years old. I was born with Hemophilia. Have you ever heard of that? It's just a fancy word that means that my blood does not form clots on its own. I get an infusion of medication to help my blood clot in case of a bleeding episode. I get hurt quite often on account of my clumsiness. Not every injury is an emergency though.

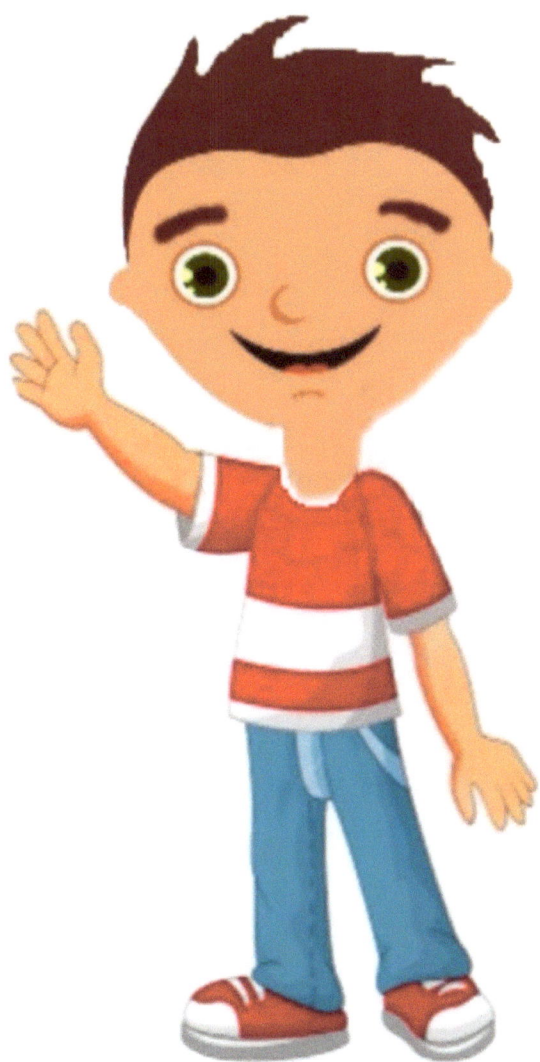

Sometimes I fall and land directly on my bottom. It's ok. My Mom and Dad just check to make sure I can walk without feeling pain and I can go right back to playing.

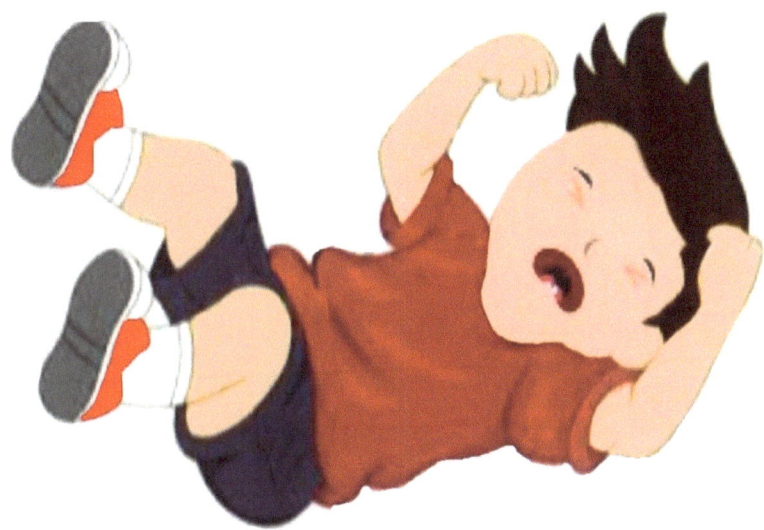

Sometimes when I am playing with my dog, she scratches me with her nails. It's ok. Mom and Dad just clean it up with soap and water and put a Band-Aid over it.

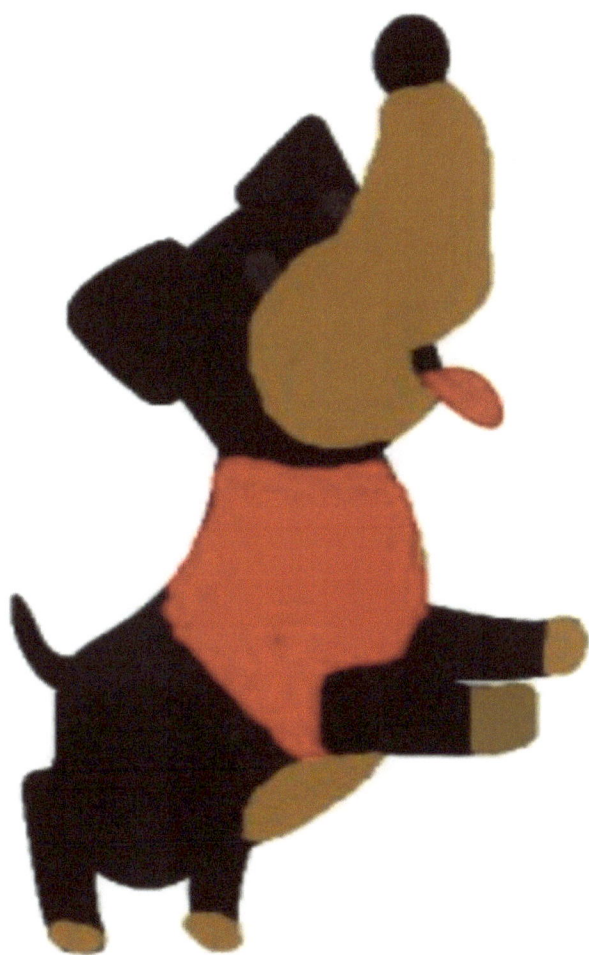

Sometimes I fall and hurt my elbow. It's ok. My Mom and Dad just put an ice pack on my elbow and check to make sure I can bend my arm without feeling pain. Afterwards, I can go right back to playing.

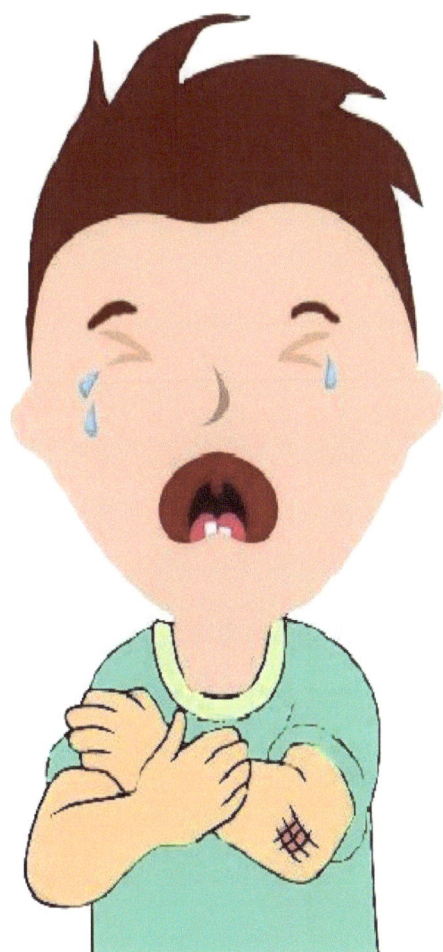

Sometimes I fall and hit my head. It's not ok. Mom and Dad give me ice to apply to the area that hurts and then they call my Hemophilia Doctor for a treatment plan. Sometimes I can get my clotting medication at home. But if it's very serious, I need to go the hospital to be sure my injury did not cause bleeding inside of my head.

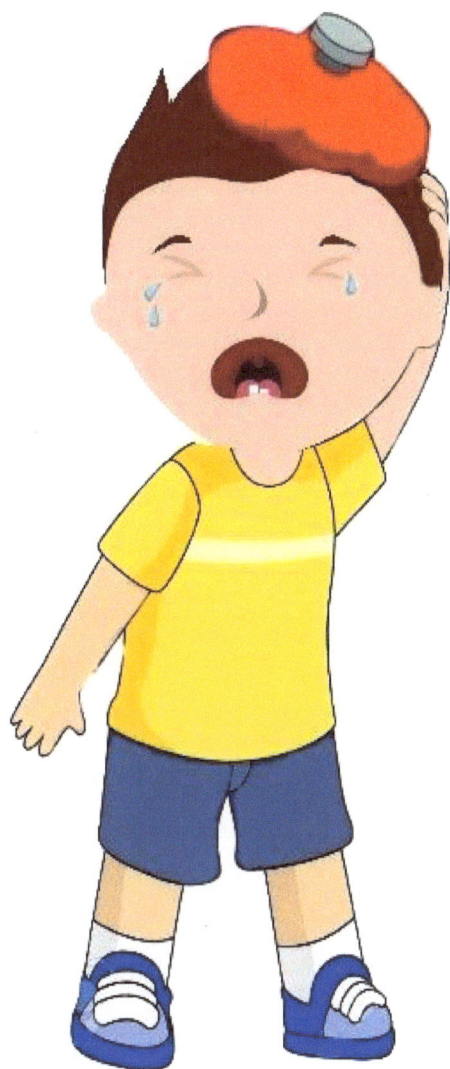

Sometimes I wake up and cannot bend my arm without feeling pain. It can be red and swollen too. It's not ok. Mom and Dad call my Hemophilia Doctor for a treatment plan. Most of the time I can get my clotting medication at home to help heal this joint or muscle bleed.

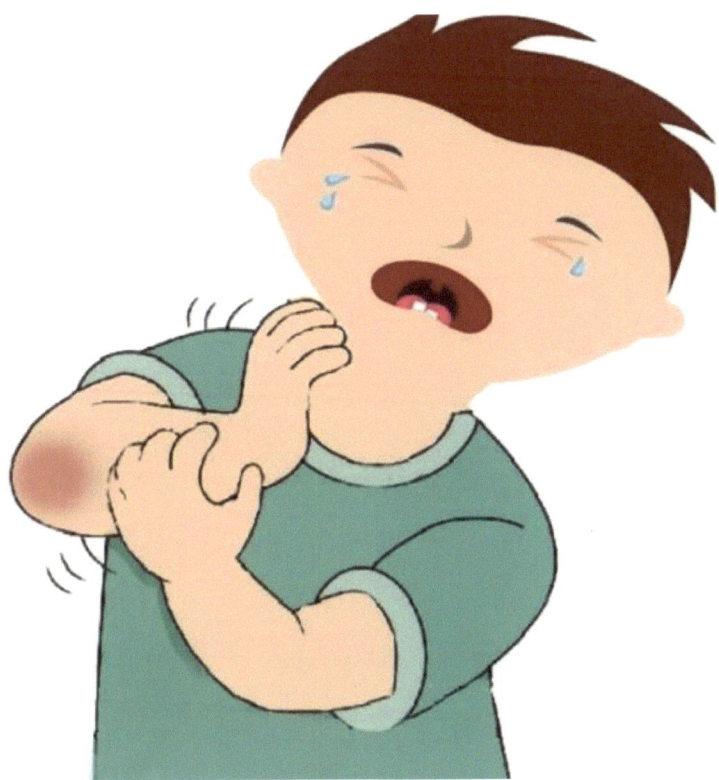

Now that you know a little bit about when it's ok and when it's not ok, let's play a game!
I'll make up a pretend injury and YOU tell me if it's ok or it's not ok, ok?

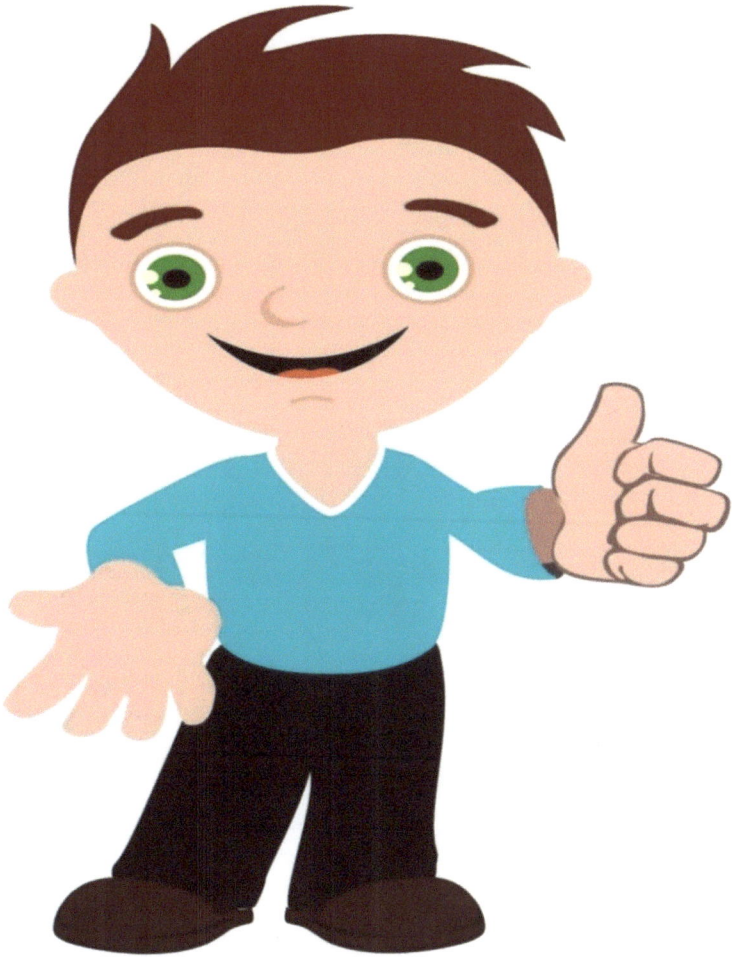

Today I fell and scraped my knee. My Mom and Dad washed it with soap and water and covered the scrape with a Band-Aid. Is this ok or not ok?

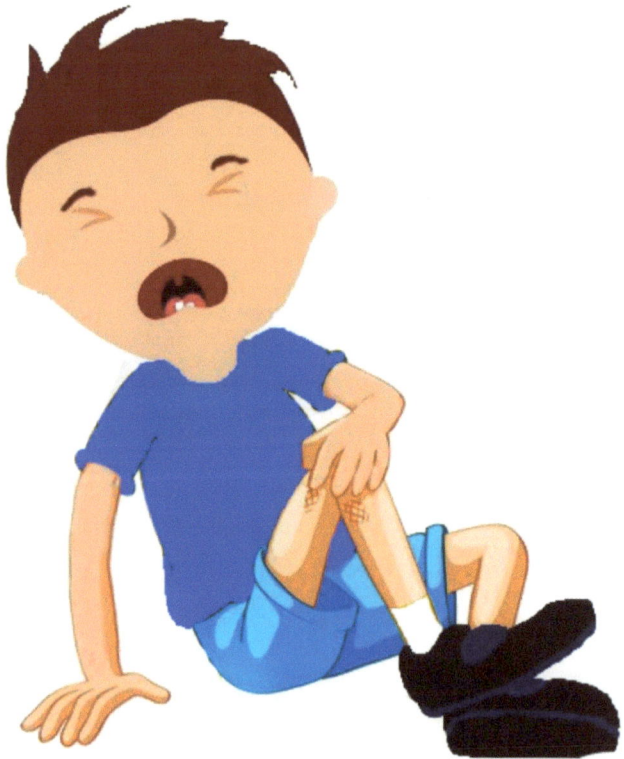

THAT'S RIGHT…IT'S OK! As long as the bleeding has stopped, *and* I can still walk and bend my leg without pain, I do not need any further treatment.

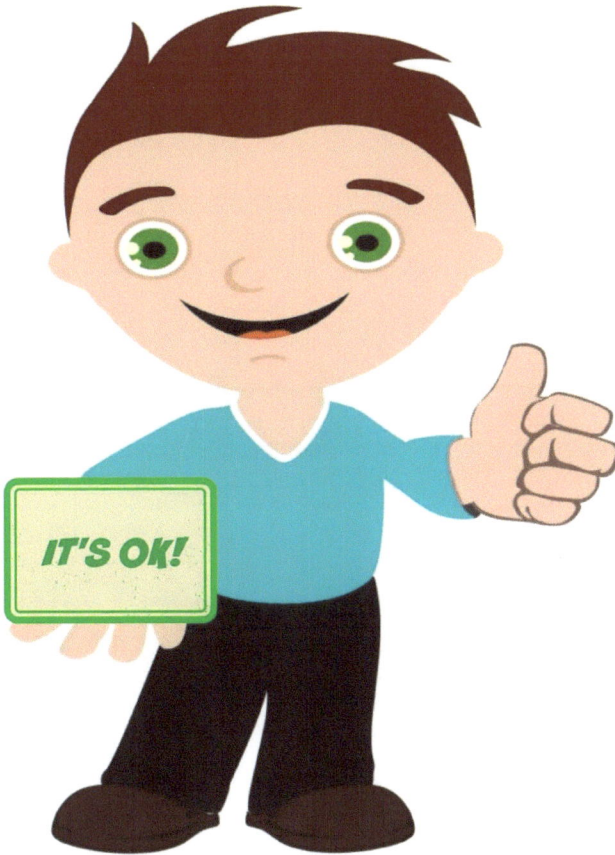

Today at school someone threw a ball and it hit me in the head. My head feels sore and I feel dizzy. Is this ok or not ok?

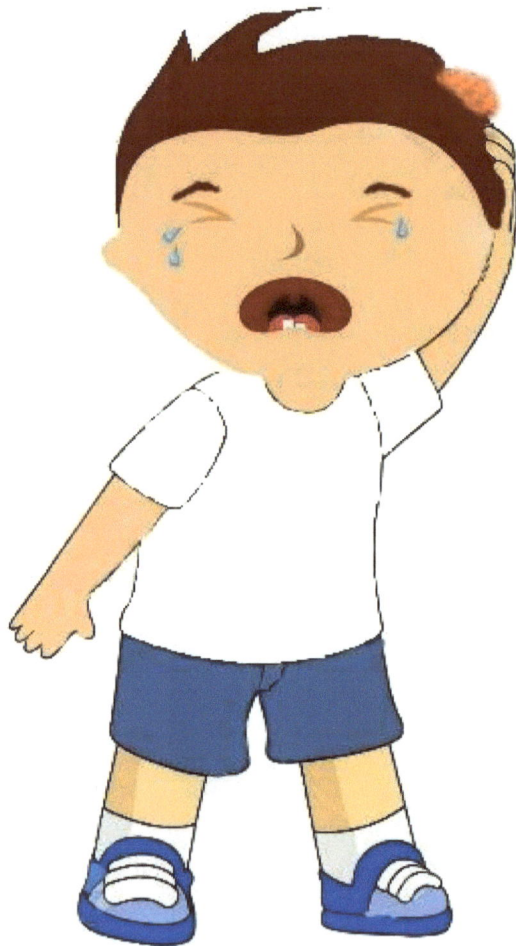

This is not ok. My teacher needs to call my Mom and Dad immediately while I put ice on my head.

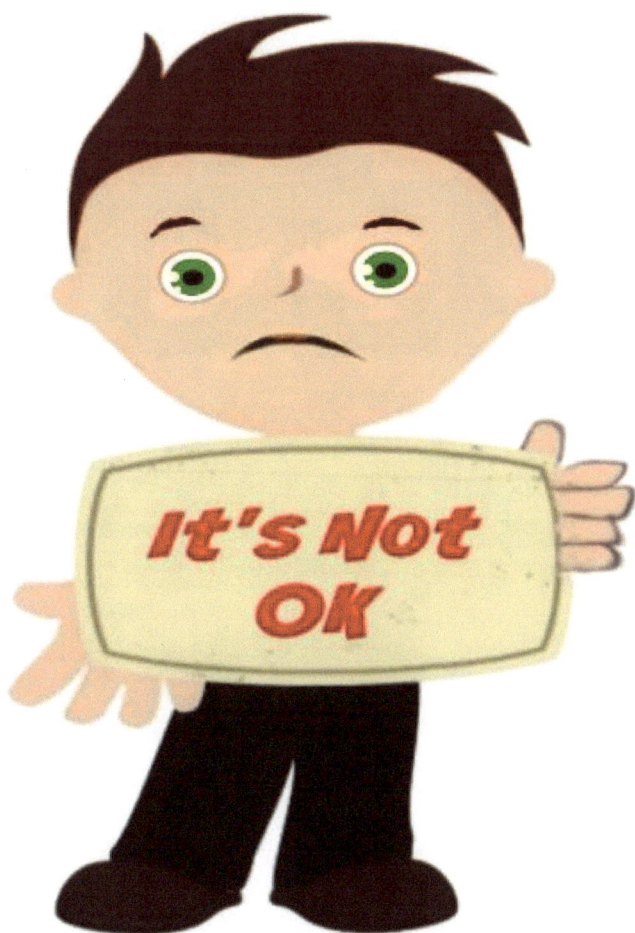

While I was brushing my teeth before bed, I noticed some blood on my toothbrush. It wasn't a lot of blood and after 15 minutes, I didn't see bleeding in my mouth anymore. Is this ok or not ok?

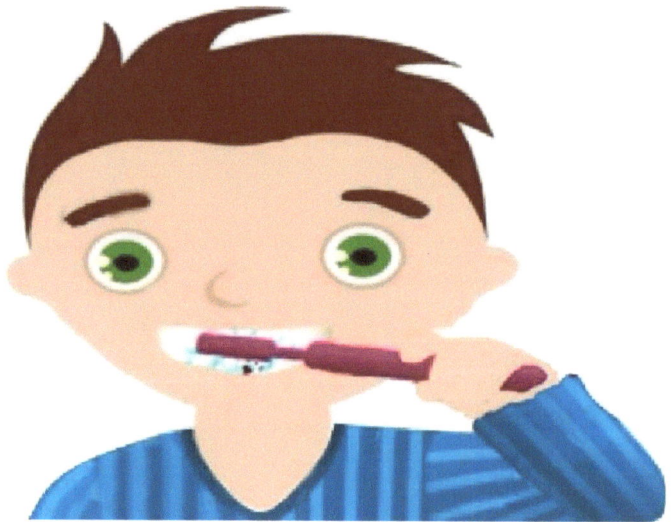

This is ok! But if my gums continued to bleed for more than 15 minutes I might have needed some clotting medication.

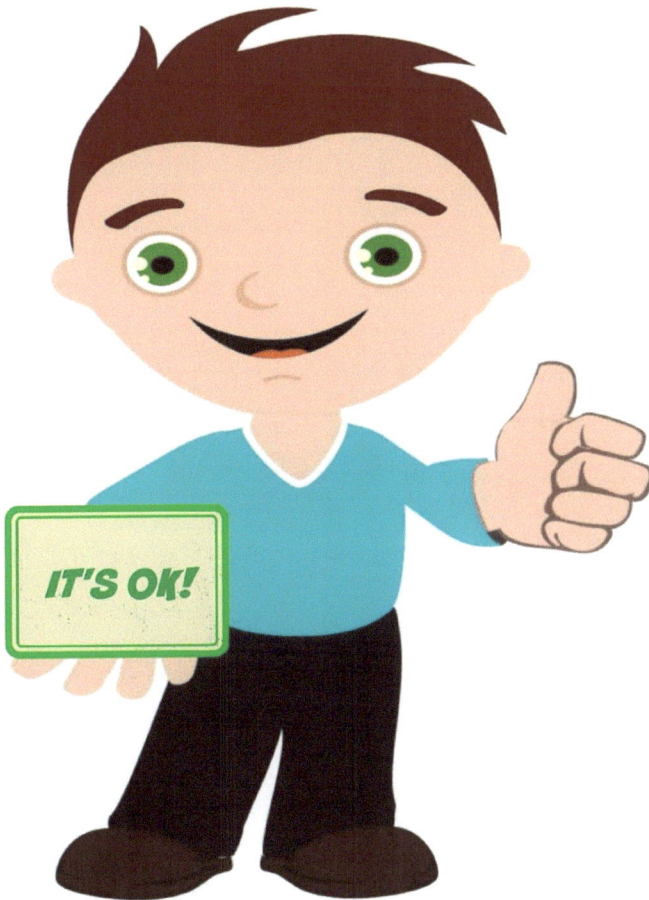

IT'S OK!

This morning when I woke up, I could not bend my leg. I looked down and my knee was swollen and red.   Is this ok or not ok?

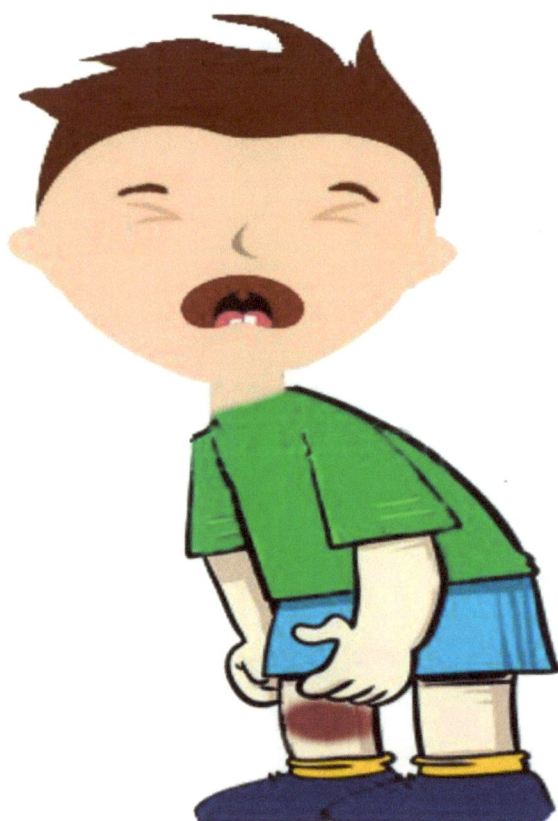

This is not ok. Most likely I am having a joint bleed and I need to ice the area while Mom or Dad call my Hemophilia Doctor for a treatment plan. I will probably receive my medication at home. I will need to continue to ice the area while I rest today.

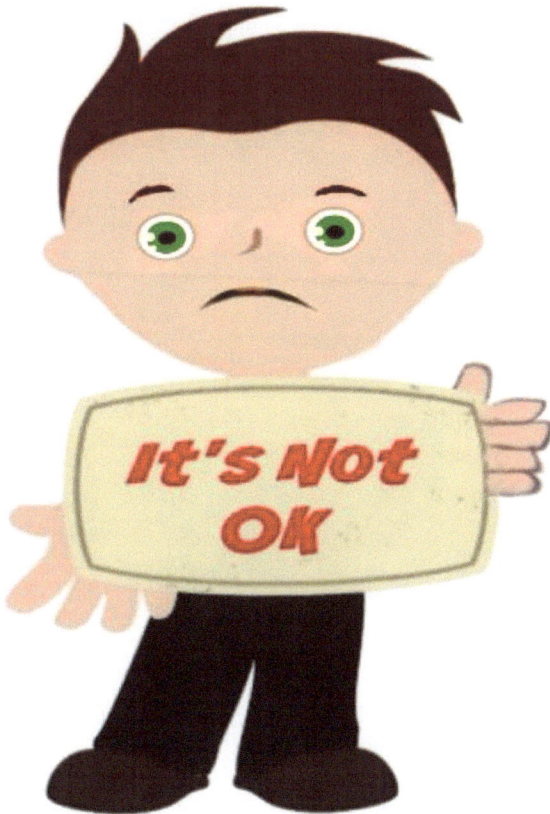

You are so smart! I'm so proud of how much you've learned.

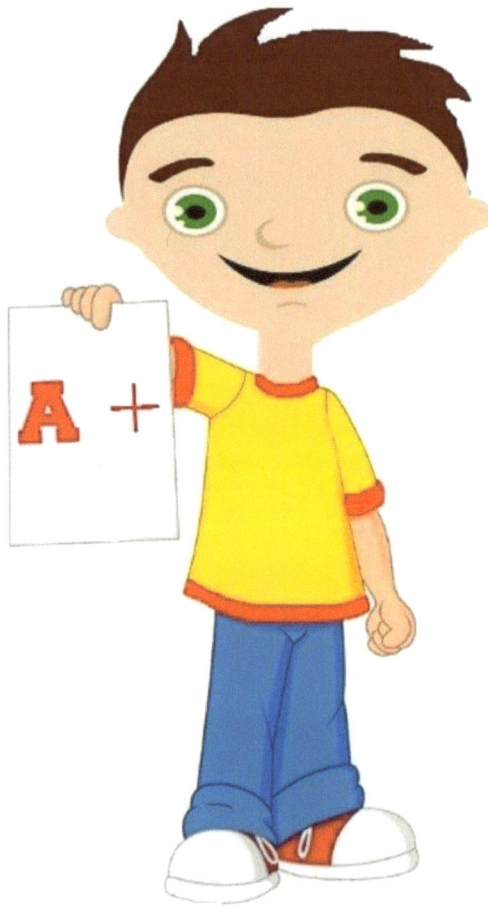

Note:

All injuries should be handled according to your own Hemophilia treatment plan. This book should not be used to determine the severity of injuries or whether injuries require treatment.

www.ingramcontent.com/pod-product-compliance
Lightning Source LLC
Chambersburg PA
CBHW041719200326
41520CB00001B/166